Weight Loss

Lose Weight Fast With 7-Day Low Carb Meal Plan

Table of contents

Introduction

It has become very fashionable in recent years to attempt to eliminate carbohydrates entirely from your diet. This is very difficult (if not almost impossible) to do – this would eliminate all fruit and vegetables from your diet, and can be extremely unhealthy. Instead, this plan will help you reduce carbohydrates and so lose weight.

It is a good idea to attempt to eliminate refined sugars and starches from your diet as far as possible, since these tend to be lacking in essential vitamins and minerals, as well as causing spikes in blood sugar which can lead to sugar cravings, making it harder to keep on track with your diet.

Fibre is an extremely important component of your diet – not only will it promote a feeling of fullness without adding extra calories, and help with digestive transit, it also slows the release of sugars into your blood. It is for this reason that you should consume whole fruit in preference for fruit juices and smoothies. Since the fibre content has been removed, the fruit sugars can enter your bloodstream at the same rate as refined sugar from a soft drink, leading to a spike in blood sugar, followed by a "crash" as your body produces insulin to store the sugar as glycogen. This crash will make you feel tired and hungry, and mean that you are triggered to eat again in order to redress your energy levels.

Look for whole fibre versions of starchy products, such as wholewheat pasta, brown rice and wholewheat bread. Even so, you should aim to consume only small amounts of these foods – the majority of your plate should be vegetables, fruit and protein.

Fat is another contentious issue – for many years the dieting industry removed fat from products in order to market them as 'healthy' and often would replace the fat with sugar in order to keep the product palatable.

The Weightwatchers points system was designed to make it easy to keep track of your calorie consumption, with a daily and weekly allowance of points. You should aim to consume 22 points per day, with a weekly addition allowance of 40 "spare" points which you can allocate as you prefer.

Whilst on the plan, all fresh fruit and vegetables (with the exception of starchy root vegetables such as potatoes and yams) have zero points, and you may consume as much as you like. (This does not apply to dried fruit however, nor to fruit juices and smoothies).

Keeping a food diary is vital while following a weight loss plan. Make sure you write down everything you consume – you may be surprised at the 'hidden' foods you consume without really noticing – biscuits at work, or a chocolate bar on your commute. It is easy to get into snacking patterns which can then become almost unnoticed, but over time will lead to weight gain. For example, if you overate by 62 calories a day (about the same calories in a custard cream biscuit) within a year you would put on six and a half pounds.

Not only will a food diary make you more aware of the foods you are consuming, it will act as a record of what you ate that week if you were more or less successful in your weight loss for that period. So, if you find one week that you have lost less than you expected, you can check back to see what you ate that week and see f you can spot the cause. Similarly, if you experienced a better than expected weight loss, you can use that week as a blueprint for other weeks. Studies have also shown that simply asked people to keep a food diary and make no other conscious changes to their diet can result in weight loss, since people are subconsciously more likely to make healthy choices under those circumstances.

You should weigh yourself once a week, and try to avoid hopping on the scales every day. Your weight can fluctuate during the day based on a variety of factors, and you should concentrate on the gradual trend of weight loss, rather than from day to day. It is also a good idea to take measurements of your waist, hip and thigh, since your proportions can change drastically with only a small adjustment to your weight. Since muscle weighs more than fat, if you exercise a lot whilst dieting it may even be possible for your weight to go up, even as your dress size shrinks.

And finally, a quick word about weight loss supplements. In every chemist, there are rows of pills claiming to 'support weight loss' and 'reduce cravings'. The vast majority of these are useless – don't waste your money.

Chapter 1 – Breakfasts

Remember that you can add fruit to all these recipes without adding additional points.

Banana Pancakes:

Makes: 12 pancakes

Points: 6 points per 2 pancakes

You will need:

2 handfuls of frozen or fresh berries – blackberries, raspberries or blueberries

2 Tablespoons oficing sugar

2 Tablespoons of self-raising flour

1 tablespoon of flax seeds

1 tablespoon oftoasted wheat germ

2 tablespoons of skimmed milk (you may need to adjust this to get the correct consistency)

3 large egg whites

1 tablespoon of walnut oil

1 teaspoon of vanilla extract

2 medium bananas, thinly sliced

A little cooking spray for frying

<u>Method:</u>

Add two squirts of cooking spray to a non-stick pan and heat over a medium flame. Meanwhile, combine the berries and sugar together in a small saucepan and heat gently, stirring from time to time. Cook until the berries begin to break down and the juice released has thickened into a syrup.

In a separate bowl, combine the flour, flax seeds, mashed banana, wheat germ, milk, egg whites, oil and vanilla extract. Beat until reasonably smooth; the mixture may still have a few small lumps in it. Don't worry about these.

Drop a tablespoon of the batter onto the hot non-stick pan and cook until bubbles start to appear. Slide a pallet knife under the pancake and flip to cook the other side.

Serve the pancakes with 2 tablespoons of syrup per serving.

Greek Style Breakfast Fritatta

This is ideal for making in advance and storing in the fridge for a quick and convenient breakfast.

Makes: 6 servings

Points: 3 per serving

You will need:

2 squirts of cooking spray

1 chopped onion

125g of fresh spinach

1 Tablespoon of roasted red peppers, diced

2 medium tomatoes, seeded and chopped

2 whole eggs, plus 9 egg whites

50g of crumbled feta cheese

2 Tablespoons of fresh herbs, such as basil, dill, etc

Salt and pepper to taste

Method:

Preheat your oven to 180 degrees. Coat an ovenproof, deep-sided dish with cooking spray and heat over a medium flame to gently soften the chopped onions. For five minutes until they are translucent. Add the peppers, spinach and tomatoes and cook until the spinach has wilted.

In a separate bowl, whisk together the eggs, egg whites, cheese herbs and seasoning. At this point, you can also add any additional flavourings (such as chilli flakes) if you desire.

Pour the egg mixture into the overproof dish and cook, stirring occasionally until the egg has begun to set. Transfer the dish to the oven and bake for around 20 minutes until the centre has set. Allow to cool and cut into wedges.

<u>**Turkey Hash and Eggs:**</u>

Makes: 4 servings

Points: 9 per serving

<u>You will need:</u>

2 squirts of cooking spray

4 medium sized raw waxy potatoes, cut into small pieces

1 onion, thinly sliced

1 Tablespoon of roasted red peppers, diced

150g of turkey pastrami, coarsely chopped

A handful of fresh cherry tomatoes

Salt and pepper

1/2 a teaspoon of rosemary, or thyme, chopped

1 Tablespoon of olive oil

4 large eggs

1 red chilli, finely sliced (optional)

<u>Method:</u>

Preheat your oven to 180 degrees. Spray an oven-proof dish or pan with cooking spray.

Parboil the potatoes in slightly salted water for six minutes or until just until fork tender. Drain and mix together with the onions, roasted peppers, pastrami, tomatoes, salt, black pepper, oil and herbsand add to the oven proof dish. Bake for about 30 to 45 minutes.

Divide the hash into four equal portions and serve with a sunny side up egg, fried with a single squirt of cooking spray.

Wholemeal Muffins with Scrambled egg and Peppers

Makes: 4 servings

Points: 5 per serving

You will Need:

2 teaspoons of olive oil

1 small raw onions, thinly sliced, or 4 spring onions, chopped

1 large green pepper, deseeded and thinly sliced

1 clove of minced garlic

4 large eggs, plus 3 egg whites

Salt and pepper

4 wholemeal muffins, toasted

Method:

Heat the oil in a nonstick pan and cook the onion and pepper until softened. Add the garlic and stir for around 30 seconds – do not allow it to burn. Turn down the heat and set the vegetables aside.

Beat together the eggs and egg whites with the salt and pepper. Scramble the eggs in the same pan, adding the vegetables back towards the end of the cooking time.

Divide the egg mixture into four, spooning onto the toasted muffins.

Maple and Cranberry Porridge:

Makes: 9 servings

Points: 6 per serving

<u>You will need:</u>

8 cups of cold water

2 cups of uncooked porridge oats

1 heaped tablespoon of dried cranberries, chopped

1 tablespoon of maple syrup

1 teaspoon of ground cinnamon

A pinch of salt

3 Tablespoons oftoasted, flaked almonds

<u>Method:</u>

The night before, combine all ingredients except the almonds in a large dish and refrigerate overnight. In the morning, heat a tablespoon of the porridge (or as much as you require) in a saucepan over a gentle heat until it is bubbling and creamy. Top with a scattering of almonds and serve.

Deviled Eggs Benedict:

Makes: 1 serving

Points: 5

<u>You will need:</u>

1 wholewheat English-style muffin

1 hard boiled egg, sliced into rounds

1 teaspoon of mustard (use smooth style rather than wholegrain)

1 Tablespoon of low-fat mayonnaise

A dash of cider vinegar

<u>Method:</u>

Cut the muffin in half and toast it. Mix together the mustard, vinegar and mayonnaise. Arrange the sliced hard boiled egg on top of each half of the muffin and pour over the sauce. Season to taste.

Greek Yoghurt To Go

Makes: 1 serving

Points: 4

<u>You will need:</u>

3 tablespoons of low-fat greek style yoghurt

A handful of grapes, cut in half lengthways

A Tablespoon of unsweetened shredded coconut

Half a small banana, sliced

A tablespoon of granola

<u>Method:</u>

In a sealable tub or clean glass jar, layer up the yoghurt with alternating layers of fruit, granola and coconut. Refrigerate until you are ready to consume it.

Chapter 2 – Lunches

<u>Roasted Vegetable Wrap:</u>

Makes: 2 servings

Points: 5 per wrap

<u>You will need:</u>

2 Tablespoons of mixed roasted vegetables – peppers, onions, courgettes and mushrooms. Roast for 45 minutes in a low oven with unpeeled cloves of garlic and a few squirts of cooking spray.

2 wholemeal tortilla wraps

2 Tablespoons of Quark

<u>Method:</u>

Warm the wraps in the microwave for a few seconds to soften them. Spread each wrap with a tablespoon each of Quark and vegetables, then roll up and eat straight away. For extra flavour, you can add some roughly torn leaves of basil, or a few slices of fresh chilli.

<u>Pasta Salad:</u>

Makes: 1 serving

Points: 4

<u>You will need:</u>

40g of dry weight wholemeal pasta – you can easily make multiple portions of this meal and save them in the fridge

5 cherry tomatoes, halved

1 spring onion, chopped

1 tablespoon of roasted red peppers

About 3 inches of cucumber, chopped into chunks and deseeded

Fresh herbs to taste

<u>Method:</u>

Cook the wholewheat pasta in slightly salted water for 10 minutes (or according to the instructions on the packet) until it is tender but still has some bite to it. Drain and allow to cool.

Mix with the other ingredients, adding salt and pepper to taste. Refrigerate until you are ready to consume it.

Onion and Potato Soup:

This is idea to make in advance and take to work for quick reheating in the microwave.

Makes: 4 servings

Points: 2 per serving

You will need:

1 small onion, chopped

5 squirts of cooking spray

300 g of raw floury potatoes, peeled and chopped

2 cloves of garlic

1 litre of chicken or vegetable stock

Salt and pepper

80 g of savoy or white cabbage, thinly shredded and with any woody stems removed.

Method:

In a medium saucepan, add the cooking spray and cook the onion until it softens. Add the potato, garlic and stock, bring to the boil and then turn down the heat. Allow it to gently simmer for 25 minutes until the potato is soft and starts to break up. At this point you can choose to blend the soup for a creamy texture, or simply leave it chunky.

Add the cabbage and heat for a few more minutes until it has softened. Taste and adjust the seasoning if required.

<u>Pitta Bread Pizza:</u>

Makes: 1

Points: 9

<u>You will need:</u>

1 wholemeal pitta

1 Tablespoon of marina sauce

Vegetables to top – sliced mushrooms, peppers, and onions

10 small black olives

50g mozzarella cheese

1 teaspoon of grated parmesan cheese

A pinch of oregano of pizza seasoning

Chilli flakes, if desired

<u>Method:</u>

Turn on your grill. Toast one side of the pitta bread, then spread the marinara sauce evenly over the untoasted side. Arrange the vegetables on the sauce and top with the cheese and herbs. Grill until the cheese bubbles.

No-Noodle Chinese Stir Fried Vegetables

Makes: 2 servings

Points: 1 per serving

You will need:

1 head of pak choy, sliced lengthways

2 tablespoons of snow or sugar snap peas

Half a small carrot, peeled, trimmed and sliced into thin shavings (a vegetable peeler is best for this)

1 tablespoon of canned bamboo shoots, drained

1 tablespoon of canned water chestnuts, drained and quartered

50g of mushrooms (shitaake is best, but you can also use chestnut or oyster)

Half a red pepper, thinly sliced

100ml of chicken or vegetable stock

1 tablespoon of soy sauce

1 clove of garlic, minced

1 teaspoon of grated fresh root ginger

Hot sauce to taste

Method:

Slice all the vegetables into even sized pieces to ensure they cook evenly. Heat a few squirts of cooking spray in a non-stick frying pan and add the mushrooms. Cook for a few minutes, then add the remaining vegetables (except the bamboo and water chestnuts) and cook, stirring briskly, until they begin to soften. Add the garlic and ginger, cook for another minute then add the vegetable or chicken stock.

Allow the stock to reduce and thicken, then add the chestnuts, bamboo and hot sauce (if using). Taste and adjust the seasoning with soy sauce before serving.

Tuna and Green Bean Salad

Makes: 1 serving

Points: 6

<u>You will need:</u>

Half a diced red onion

A few cherry tomatoes, halved

The juice of half a lemon

1 teaspoon of olive oil

2 teaspoons of tomato puree

A handful of cooked and halved green beans

1 teaspoon of capers

120g of canned, drained mixed beans

56g tin of tuna, drained (choose the variety which has been canned in spring water, rather than oil)

Mixed salad leaves

Salt and pepper

<u>Method:</u>

In the bottom of the bowl you intend to serve the salad in, whisk together the oil, tomato puree, lemon juice and capers. Add the beans and toss to coat thoroughly. Add the rest of the ingredients, topping with the tuna and season to taste.

Smoked Mackerel and Cous Cous

Makes: 1 serving

Points: 9

<u>You will need:</u>

40g of dry wholewheat couscous

1 orange

1 spring onion, chopped

1 carrot, peeled and grated

3 inches of cucumber, chopped

1 fillet (around 55g) of flaked smoked mackerel

A handful of watercress

<u>Method:</u>

Add the zest and juice of half the orange to the dry couscous and cover with boiling water. Allow to stand for ten minutes than fluff with a fork.

Meanwhile, slice the remaining half of the orange and combine with the other ingredients, except the watercress. Add in the cooked cous cous and serve with the fresh watercress.

Chapter 4 – Dinners

<u>**Crunchy Green Prawns**</u>

Makes: 4 servings

Points: 4 per serving

<u>You will need:</u>

1 bunch of fresh parsley, chopped

1 bunch of fresh basil, chopped

2 cloves of garlic, finely chopped or minced

Salt and pepper to taste

750g of fresh, raw, peeled prawns with the veins removed

<u>Method:</u>

For the marinade, mix together the chopped herbs with the garlic, oil, salt and pepper in a large, sealable plastic bag. Add the prawns to the marinade and squeeze and mix the bag to make sure that each prawn is completely coated in the marinade. Leave the prawns in the fridge for a minimum of one hour, up to overnight.

Coat a griddle pan with some low-fat cooking spray. Heat the pan to medium and tip in enough of the prawns to cover the bottom of the pan in a single layer (you will have to do this in batches to avoid overcrowding the pan). Cook the prawns for around three minutes on each side, or until they turn pink and are cooked through. Serve with a fresh green salad.

Aubergine Curry

Makes: 4 servings

Points: 5 per serving

<u>You will need:</u>

1 small aubergine, sliced and cut into centimeter cubes

A quarter of a head of cauliflower, divided into bite sized florets

1 jar of reduced calorie Jalfreezi sauce (or other curry sauce of your choosing)

400g can of chickpeas, drained

A small bunch of fresh coriander, leaves and stalks chopped1

<u>Method:</u>

Preheat your oven to 180 degrees. Line a baking sheet with foil and spread out the aubergine and cauliflower in a single layer. Mist with a couple of squirts of low-calorie cooking spray and roast for 25 minutes, turning once, until the vegetables have started to brown and soften.

Pour the curry sauce into a pan and heat with the chickpeas on a medium heat. Add the roasted vegetables and simmer for ten minutes. Scatter with the chopped coriander before serving.

Feta and Lamb Burgers:

Makes: 1 serving

Points: 9

<u>You will need:</u>

100g lean minced lamb

1 clove of garlic, crushed

A sprig of chopped fresh rosemary

Half a teaspoon of dried oregano

25g of feta, crumbled

Salt and pepper

<u>Method:</u>

Mix the ingredients together thoroughly – it is easiest to do this with your hands. Shape into a round and grill under a medium heat until the outside of the burger is well coloured and the inside is cooked through. Serve with salad leaves and fresh tomatoes.

Shape into a patty. Grill the burger until cooked through.

<u>Steak with Grilled Vegetables:</u>

Makes: 1 serving

Points: 7

<u>You will need:</u>

1 courgette, sliced into rounds

1 red pepper, sliced and deseeded

5 spears of asparagus

1 clove of garlic

1 teaspoon of olive oil

1 teaspoon of balsamic vinegar

1 sprig of fresh rosemary, chopped

150g fillet steak

<u>Method:</u>

Toss the sliced courgette, pepper and asparagus spears in the binegar and half the olive oil. Season and arrange in a single layer on a baking sheet under a hot grill, checking and turning regularly.

Brush the steak with the remaining olive oil and rub in the chopped fresh rosemary on each side.

Heat a griddle pan until it smokes and cook the steak to your preferred level of pinkness. Serve with the vegetables and some fresh cherry tomatoes.

Pasta de Mare:

Makes: 1 serving

Points: 10

You will need:

1 sliced red onion

Half a tin of chopped tomatoes

1 teaspoon of olive oil

A pinch of chilli powder (adjust to personal taste)

60g of dried tagliatelle

Salt and pepper

100g of cooked mixed seafood (prawns, mussels, calamari, etc)

2 teaspoons of grated parmesan cheese

Method:

Cook the pasta according to the package instructions. Slice the red onion and fry in the oil for a few minutes until softened, then add the tomatoes and chilli, if using. Simmer for ten minutes until the sauce begins to thicken.

Add the seafood to the sauce and allow to heat through. Stir in the cooked pasta, ensuring that each strand is evenly coated with the sauce, scatter with the parmesan and serve.

Pesto Chicken:

Makes: 1 serving

Points: 8

<u>You will need:</u>

1 skinless chicken breast

1 teaspoon of olive oil

1 Tablespoon of crème fresh

1 Tablespoon of pesto

A handful of cherry tomatoes

The juice of half a lemon

A small bunch of fresh basil

<u>Method:</u>

With a sharp knife, butterfly the chicken breast so that it cooks more quickly, and pan-fry for around twenty minutes in the oil, or until cooked through. A few minutes before the end of the cooking time, add the cherry tomatoes to the pan.

Meanwhile, mix together the crème fresh, pesto and lemon juice. Use the sauce to top the cooked chicken breast and scatter with the torn basil leaves before serving. Serve with a mixed leaf salad.

Baked Mediterranean Cod with Pasta:

Makes: 1 serving

Points: 8

<u>You will need:</u>

200g tin of chopped tomatoes

2 teaspoons of tomato purée

1 clove of garlic, chopped

A few fresh thyme leaves

1 tablespoon of balsamic vinegar

1 teaspoon of capers

5 pitted black olives

125g skinless cod fillet

40g dried tagliatelle

A few leaves of fresh basil

<u>Method:</u>

In a pan, heat the chopped tomatoes, tomato purée, garlic and thyme leaves for ten minutes until they start to thicken. Pour the sauce into a small, ovenproof dish along with the balsamic vinegar, capers and black olives. Place the cod fillet on top and bake at 180 degrees for 15 minutes.

Will the cod is in the oven, cook the pasta according to the package instructions. Serve with a few fresh basil leaves.

Chapter 4 – Desserts and Sweets

<u>Marshmallow Chocolate Fudge</u>

Makes: 36 pieces

Points: 3 per piece

<u>You will need:</u>

300g caster sugar

150ml fat-free evaporated milk

2 tablespoons of margarine

300g dark chocolate

14 large marshmallows

<u>Method:</u>

Coat an 8x8-inch pan with cooking spray and line with baking parchment. Combine the sugar, margarine and evaporated milk in a small saucepan, bring to the boil and then turn the heat down. Allow it to bubble gently for three minutes.

Cut the chocolate into chunks, then stir into the evaporated milk along with the marshmallows. The pan should not be on the heat for this – the residual heat will be enough to melt the chocolate. Stir until smooth and completely combined.

Pour the mixture into your prepared pan and smooth the top. Refrigerate for at least two hours, or until firm, then carefully divide it into six rows and columns to make 36 squares.

<u>**Lemon Bars**</u>

Makes: 24 bars

Points: 3 per bar

<u>You will need:</u>

300g plain flour

5 tablespoons of light soft brown sugar

8 tablespoons of cold butter, cut into chunks

4 large eggs

A dash of vanilla extract (do not use synthetic vanilla flavouring)

300g icing sugar (divided)

The juice of two lemons

<u>Method:</u>

Preheat your oven to 170 degrees. Line an oven proof dish with baking parchment.

Make your pie crust by combining the flour and butter in a food processor until the mixture resembles coarse breadcrumbs. Press the crust into the prepared dish in an even layer and bake in the over for 20 minutes until it has turned a light golden brown.

While it is cooking, mix beat the eggs in a large bowl until they are frothy, then add the vanilla and 200g of the icing sugar. Mix well, then add the lemon juice and remaining sugar.

When the pie crust is cooked, remove it from the oven and turn the oven down to 160 degrees. Pour the lemon mixture into the still-warm crust and return to the oven for half an hour. Allow to cool before cutting into bars.

Amaretto and Plum Pudding

Makes: 6 servings

Points: 4 per serving

You will need:

450g of fresh, pitted plums, cut into quarters

4 tablespoons of almond liqueur

110g of plain flour

A pinch of salt

1 medium egg

300ml of skimmed milk

1 teaspoon of vanilla extract

1 teaspoon of caster sugar

1 level teaspoons of icing sugar

A few squirts of calorie controlled cooking spray,

Method:

Allow the plums to soak in the almond liqueur for at least half an hour, stirring occasionally. Preheat the oven to 180 degrees and coat a shallow, ovenproof dish with cooking spray.

Meanwhile, beat together the caster sugar, flour, salt, milk, egg and vanilla extract. Drain the plums but do not discard the liquid and add to the baking tray. Pour over the cake batter and bake for 25 minutes, or until set and golden.

Serve the pudding with the reserved liqueur as a sauce.

Chapter 5 – Sides and Snacks

<u>One Point Coleslaw</u>

Makes: 4 servings

Points: 1 per serving

<u>You will need:</u>

200g of raw cabbage, finely shredded with any large woody stalks removed

2 spring onions, finely sliced

2 tablespoons of low fat mayonnaise

A dash of garlic salt and cayenne pepper, Tabasco or Sriracha sauce

A squeeze of lemon juice

Salt and pepper

A quarter of a teaspoon of celery seeds

<u>Method:</u>

Combine all ingredients well until the cabbage is thoroughly coated. Refrigerate until you are ready to serve.

<u>Crispy Courgette Fries:</u>

Makes: 4 servings

Points: 3 per serving

<u>You will need:</u>

2 medium courgettes, cut lengthways into four and then halved to make eight lengths per courgette

50g plain four

1 tablespoons of panko breadcrumbs

2 egg whites, beaten until frothy

1 teaspoon of italian seasoning or oregano

A pinch of salt

A few squirts of low-fat cooking spray

<u>Method:</u>

Preheat your oven to 190 degrees. In one bowl, combine the flour, salt and seasoning, and in another place the panko breadcrumbs. Dredge each piece of courgette in the flour, then dip into the egg whites and then roll in the panko breadcrumbs. Arrange the courgettes on a lined baking sheet and spray with the low-fat cooking spray. Cook for ten minutes or until crisp, turning occasionally.

Chinese Style Chicken Legs

Makes: 6 servings (2 legs = 1 serving)

Points: 5 per serving

You will need:

12 chicken legs, skins removed

8 spring onions, chopped

2 teaspoons of sesame seeds

For the marinade:

2 tablespoons each of barbecue sauce, soy sauce, oyster sauce and clear honey

1 teaspoon of chilli paste (adjust the heat to personal taste)

2 cloves of minced garlic

2 teaspoons of minced fresh root ginger

Method:

Preheat your oven to 180 degrees. For ease of cleanup you can line a large baking sheet with foil, or use a disposable foil tray.

Combine the marinade ingredients in a large bowl or ziplock plastic bag. Add the spring onions and chicken legs, and mix to coat them.

Tip the chicken out into a large baking tray (the legs should form a single layer to ensure the cook evenly) and soon over and remaining marinade. Cover the baking sheet with aluminium foil and cook for twenty minutes. Remove the foil and continue to cook, occasionally spooning the sauce over the chicken and turning them.

Check that the chicken is cooked all the way through (the flesh should be opaque, firm and piping hot) and sprinkle with sesame seeds before serving. If in doubt, a meat thermometer is a useful gadget to have in the kitchen, and will ensure that your meat is always cooked thoroughly.

Tip: these chicken legs are ideal to have cold as a high protein snack. Simply keep them refrigerated before you eat them.

<u>Really Quick Treats:</u>

1 Jaffa Cake –1 Point per biscuit

1 Crumpet – 2 Points per crumpet

6 Almonds – 2 Points

1 Apple – 0 Points

1 Hard boiled egg – 2 Points

10 olives – 1 point (only for olives in brine, not oil)

Conclusion

We hope you have enjoyed this guide to low-carb weight loss recipes. Losing weight can be tricky, and it is easy to become discouraged. But remind yourself that the goal is sustainable weight loss, not a "quick fix" or magic solution. In the long run, weight which is lost quickly is often regained just as fast, and your should be aiming to make long-term, sustainable changes to your diet and exercise habits.

Portion control is extremely important – it is very easy to lose sight of what a 'normal' sized portion looks like. Restaurants and cookery shows often serve portions which are very large – this is fine for a treat or a special meal out, but it should not become the 'usual' size for every day consumption. These large portion sizes encourage the diner to keep eating even after their stomach is full. Over time, it gets easier and easier to ignore the signals from your brain that your stomach is full, and overeating becomes more and more ingrained.

Many people who are considering going on a diet for weight loss are concerned that they will be 'hungry all the time'. This should not be the case, but it is good to relearn what true stomach-hunger feels like. This is separate from cravings which can be connected to habit, boredom, emotions or pleasure. If you try to eat only from hunger, it becomes easier to stop when you are full, even if there is food on your plate. Many people are told as children to finish everything that it in front of them, and this is not a good habit to carry over into adult life.

www.ingramcontent.com/pod-product-compliance
Lightning Source LLC
Chambersburg PA
CBHW050804240726
48654CB00008B/622